My Childs's Mental Health

All You Want To Know About Children's Mental State

Kristy J. King

Table Of Contents

Presentation

It is routinely less requesting recognizing the physical needs of a child when it comes to endeavoring to allow palatably nutritious food, water, warmth, and so on.

When it comes to the mental well-being of a child, the parent may not have such basic time at all.

A child's mental strong may not be as self-evident as his or her physical condition or needs, hence their parent would have to be learned on the subject of mental well-being advancement sometime recently endeavoring to urge the child's advance.

Get all the data you'd like here. My Childs's Mental Well-being What You Want To Know Nearly Children's Mental State

Chapter One
Children's Mental Well-being

The perfect great mental well-being condition would be where the child can think clearly in social settings and learn modern abilities to adjust to the encompassing needs of the time and to moreover be comfortable with creating his or her claim self-certainty, tall self-regard and a sincerely solid viewpoint in life.

 The **Essentials** Within the journey to get it and give well for the child's ideal mental development, the parent should be able to supply components such as unrestricted cherish from the family individuals, educating the child on self-certainty and tall self-regard measures, investing as much time as conceivable with the child to energize social interaction and development so that the child will be comfortable in knowing how to amplify the same to other unused augmentations at whatever point and wherever presented.

By taking the time to connect more with the child through play and other implies of interaction, the parent will also be able to empower the child to memorize how to acknowledge direction and supportive gestures from other sources such as instructors and steady caregivers.

It'll too offer assistance to the child to distinguish secure and secure encompassing in which to associate with others.

With suitable direction and teaching, the child will be able to form all the different choices required for ideal mental well-being development.

Chapter Two
Supporting Inspiration And Certainty

Self-regard cases are regularly associated with the thought handle that this is an imperative fixing in advancing the perfect development of a child's positive and sure deportment and viewpoint.

This will too be the contributing calculate to the mental development and comparing social flexibility of the child.

Self-Worth is One of the most commitments a parent can make to creating this in a child's developing handle would be to guarantee there's moreover of positive sustaining styles utilizing adore, care, and regard as the premise of making a sure and agreeable child.

When a child is instructed to see themselves and learn to acknowledge and like what they see gazing back at them, at that point ,the street to learning certainty will be built up.

Making the child get how vital it is to be able to accept themselves and as it selects positive enhancements to create a positive requirement for changes ought to be a portion of the sustaining handle given by the parent.

It is imperative to continuously take the time and inconvenience to fortify the got to construct a strong self-certainty demeanor within the child, and this will be done with a parcel of positive comments and supportive gestures.

From indeed as early as the earliest stages arrange, the small one will be able to see its self-worth when fitting reactions are given to its different distinctive cries.

In receiving this consideration at whatever point the child cries out for it.

The primary steps to building certainty will be made.

 Although at this point, the infant truly does not realize the suggestions to its mental development.

Children as well will inevitably capture on to this as they learn how to do things agreeing to what is satisfactory and in this way appreciate the coming about positive support and laud that will offer assistance to also construct their certainty levels.

Chapter Three
Recognize Changed Behavior In Your Child

Each parent got to be concerned with any changes in behavior design a child may appear as these appear to donate essential data to the parent on what is going on within the child's judgment skills and in this way his or her world.

What Is unmistakable there are many benefits in being able to recognize these changes and this capacity to examine the changes in a few cases is because it infers a parent has got to assist in how to handle a particular circumstance.

Most restorative specialists will confirm the truth that a child's essential appearance of a particular behavior is as a run the show formed by interfacing various more diminutive behaviors.

Contrasting the child adapt to or appreciate a particular circumstance would offer assistance, especially if the parent was able to precisely recognize the behavioral plan, in this way enabling the parent to provide the correct comparing offer assistance to the child.

In endeavoring to urge it to the child, the parent would get to unmistakably observe the diverse reactions and appearance of sentiments as this will about ceaselessly illustrate the child's thought to plan for needs subsequently contributing to a conceivable more uniform set of behavioral affinity that can be more easily examined.

The child will as well learn to utilize the parent as their essential case by observing the parents' particular responses and behavioral plan and in a couple of cases choosing to imitate these with as numerous resemblances as conceivable.

Hence the parent would get to be exceptionally cautious in how they appear they have behavioral plans as they should be persistently careful of the children's capabilities and understanding levels of imitating such appearance.

Through such discernments, the parent will be able to prevalent cope with the unmistakable varieties such as a strong will child, a child that must be competitive persistently, a child that needs a portion of back, and give the comparing lessons as required.

Chapter Four
Nearly Birth Absconds

All guardians are concerned with the diverse perspectives of the children and this, oftentimes than not begins right from the time of conception, and as a run, the show, never closes.

Perhaps one of the essential concerns would be around any conceivable birth absconds that a child may be born with and how to oversee as best as conceivable should this be the case.

What Can Happen Birth surrenders are more regularly than not characterized as any winning variations from the norm of structure, work, or body assimilation framework that will or may not be self-evident at the time of the birth.

For the more self-evident irregularities, the imperative supporting groups will be able to assist the parent in either learning how to oversee the birth defect or offer help to the parent explore all choices available in case any, to correct the deformation as some time recently long since it is sensible.

The assistant or metabolic forsakes would be centered basically on specific body parts that are either lost or distorted in a couple of ways which may be caused by a couple of issues with the body chemistry that was unable for many reasons to create a add up to and idealize child inside the womb.

These forsake more frequently than not join cases of spina bifida, cleft sense of taste, clubfoot and inborn isolated hip, and various other conceivable results.

The forsakes caused by the intrinsic contaminations can more frequently than not result in inconsistencies when the mother experience defilement at some point as of late or during the pregnancy organize.

These contaminations will cause birth surrenders and can be inside the outline of rubella, cytomegalovirus, syphilis, toxoplasmosis, Venezuelan equine encephalic, parvovirus, and chicken pox.

The pregnancy period is usually organized where security measures got to be taken to control the chances of the mother having to oversee the invasion of terminates that might have especially harmful impacts on the developing life.

Shockingly this closeness of twisting isn't continuously due to some contaminations as in fact strong guardians, are a few of the time shown with a child with clear distortions.

Chapter Five
About behavioral obstacles

All children at one time or another have some form of behavior problem.

This is largely an acceptable standard that most guardians can oversee.

In any event, when a particular plan of behavior becomes unrelenting and harmful, public assistance should be arranged to understand and adjust the circumstances so that all parties can monitor it.

The most common behavioral obstacles that don't impair or unreasonably hurt would include overactive children getting into dangerous situations, mischief, sometimes rebelliousness, and other behaviors.

Other gentler behavior plans. In any case, when these softer notions take on a more genuine and depraved negative appearance at this stage, they cannot be regarded as common but must be considered directly as behavioral disturbances.

The most common warning signs of such negatives and often dangerous behavior are injuring or harming yourself, pets, or others, looking at or spraying property, lying or appropriating, academic failure and inevitably truancy, early smoking, drinking, and drug use, early sexual development, a crisis of visitation and debate, and contracting vibrations for the main characters.

Whatever happens will inevitably be a problem for the child, and parents will always feel confused as how to supervise in such cases.

The confusion and shock that both parties feels must be appropriately monitored so that progress, can be made in accepting and overcoming this negativity and offering support.

The child recognizes the idea of offering help to bring about calmer, better behavior that others can live with.

Subsequent investigations, were able to show that it was not constant external circumstances that contributed to negative behavioral plans, but in some cases, possibly some blockages within the brain.

Claims for certain chemicals or the bulky nature of chemicals inside the brain could be one of the causes of experienced behavior, so they should explore that confidence as well.

Chapter Six
Mental Wellbeing Diversions For Children

Working with children with mental well-being issues can be very challenging and, including this would be the complication that most of these children would not be willing and open to the assistance being given due to their mental condition.

Subsequently, utilizing recreations as an invigorating calculation would be a great and empowering device, to begin with.

Tips that these recreations can effortlessly be sourced and

acquired online or at any amusement store.

Due to the assortment available, the parent would get to consider the child's mental condition and what it would take to fortify it the perfect way the most perfect way conceivable.

It isn't continuously essential to purchase these recreations as a few can be high quality or development fair from a few instinctive creative energy to suit the wants at hand.

Board and card diversions are, as a rule, a great way to fortify the intellect.

These boards' diversions are, as a rule particularly planned to address the mental well-being issues the child may be confronting such as sadness, self-regard issues, consideration shortage hyperactivity clutter, and numerous more.

These board diversions can too be utilized from a helpful point that would empower the child to be included without being forced to confront the genuine mental well-being condition head-on.

It can too contribute to helping the child hone progress of the social aptitudes that most mental well-being risky children bashfully absent from.

This will too inevitably offer assistance to progress the self-regard issues the child may be going through.

The parent can utilize conventional recreations with the included, include getting the child to form one positive explanation approximately themselves each turn they play.

Methodology diversions can too be especially valuable devices as they too help to construct the self-confidence of the child amid the course of making strides on issue

understanding aptitude and progressing on working as a group.

Chapter Eight
Make sure to take care of yourself

Exercise should be in the form of walking, running, cycling, and swimming.

However, don't run as it'll strain your joints, especially the knees, If you're over fifty.

Swimming is a stylish form of exercise for all periods and you can do it at any time of the day.

An hour of swimming is enough.

It takes you too

Our bodies need a certain quantum of rest each day.

When you have children with you, you'll find yourself veritably fluently tired because you have to take care of your baby to eat, be safe, and get enough rest.

You'll stay overall hours to take care of the baby.

 All this conditioning will leave you exhausted.

Try to get enough rest whenever possible.

Indeed half an hour of sleep is good for you.

 Another factor in maintaining a healthy mind and body is proper nutrition.

You need to make sure you get all your nutrients in the form of vitamins, fiber, carbohydrates, and protein in balanced reflections and supplements.

These foods and supplements will ensure your body gets what it needs, thereby keeping your mind healthy and clear.

Wrap

To give your child the best possible mental and physical health care, you need to be in good physical and mental health to do so.

When you are not one hundred percent, your mental and physical mindset will not be able to track and catch any deviations in your child's ability to be physically and mentally sociable.

This is why it's so important to have a proper regimen of exercise, rest, and nutrition to maintain good physical and mental well-being.